The Complete Keto Chaffle Recipes Cookbook:

The most-wanted recipes cookbook with easy and detailed instructions. Stay fit and burn fat in a few steps.

SARAH BUCKLEY

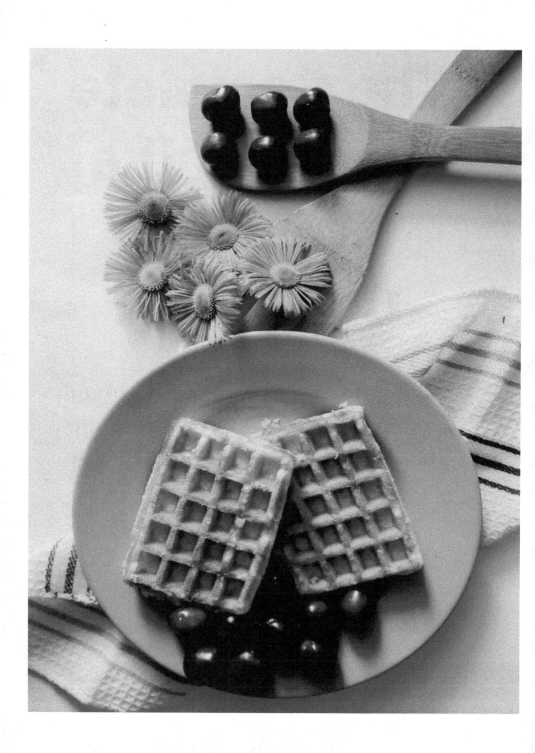

Legal & Disclaimer

The information contained in this book and its contents is not designed to replace or take the place of any form of medical or professional advice; and is not meant to replace the need for independent medical, financial, legal or other professional advice or services, as may be required. The content and information in this book have been provided for educational and entertainment purposes only.

The content and information contained in this book have been compiled from sources deemed reliable, and it is accurate to the best of the Author's knowledge, information, and belief. However, the author cannot guarantee its accuracy and validity and cannot be held liable for any errors and/or omissions. Further, changes are periodically made to this book as and when needed. Where appropriate and/or necessary, you must consult a professional (including but not limited to your doctor, attorney, financial advisor or such other professional advisor) before using any of the suggested remedies, techniques, or information in this book.

Upon using the contents and information contained in this book, you agree to hold harmless the Author from and against any damages, costs, and expenses, including any legal fees potentially resulting from the application of any of the information provided by this

TABLE OF CONTENTS

TABLE OF CONTENTS 5

INTRODUCTION 9

How to Make Chaffles? 10

11 Tips to Make Chaffles 11

SIMPLE CHAFFLES.......................14

1. Mayonnaise & Cream Cheese Chaffles...........................14

2. Blue Cheese Chaffle Bites.................................16

3. Raspberries Chaffles..17

4. Simple Chaffle Toast.......................................19

5. Savory Beef Chaffle.......................................20

6. Chaffles With Almond Flour 22

7. Nutter Butter Chaffles 24

8. Keto Reuben Chaffles 26

9. Carrot Chaffle Cake......................................28

10. Colby Jack Slices Chaffles 30

BREAKFAST CHAFFLE RECIPE.31

11. Crispy Chaffles With Egg & Asparagus 31

12. Delicious Raspberries taco Chaffles 33

13. Coconut Chaffles 35

14. Garlic and Parsley Chaffles 37

15. Scrambled Eggs on A Spring Onion Chaffle 39

16. Egg on A Cheddar Cheese Chaffle 42

17. Avocado Chaffle Toast 44

18. Cajun & Feeta Chaffles 46

19. Crispy Chaffles With Sausage 48

20. Chili Chaffle 50

BASIC CHAFFLES 52

21. White Bread Keto Chaffle 52

22. Cranberry and Brie Chaffle 54

23. Banana Foster Chaffle 56

24. Flaxseed Chaffle 59

25. Hazelnut Chaffle 61

26. Maple Pumpkin Chaffle 63

27. Nutty Chaffles 65

28. Crispy Chaffle With Everything but The Bagel
Seasoning 66

29. Strawberry and Cream Cheese Low-Carb Keto Waffles 68

30. Pumpkin Chaffle With Cream Cheese Glaze 70

31. Crunch Cereal Cake Chaffle 72

SWEET CHAFFLES 74

32. Spiced Pumpkin Chaffles 74

33. Vanilla Chaffle 76

34. Banana Nut Chaffle 78

35. Chocolaty Chips Pumpkin Chaffles 80

36. Oreo Chaffles 82

37. Whipping Cream Pumpkin Chaffles 84

38. Chocolate Vanilla Chaffles 86

39. Churro Waffles 87

40. Chocolate Chips Lemon Chaffles 89

SAVORY CHAFFLES RECIPES 91

41. Vegan Chaffle 91

42. Lemony Fresh Herbs Chaffles 93

43. Italian Seasoning Chaffles 95

44. Basil Chaffles 97

45. Bacon Chaffles 98

46. Sausage Chaffles..100

47. Scallion Cream Cheese Chaffle 102

48. Broccoli Chaffles..103

49. Chicken Taco Chaffles 105

50. Bacon & 3-cheese Chaffles..106

CONCLUSION............................. 108

INTRODUCTION

W hether you're looking to lose some weight or you need to burn fat, you can use the keto chaffle in your diet plan. Keto chaffle is a dietary supplement, with no calories or carbs. It contains low carbs and low calories as well. A keto chaffle is designed to help with weight loss.

How it works: the chaffle is made up of shredded coconut and pumpkin seeds. It works by providing a low-calorie carb source that provides energy to your body while keeping your blood sugar stable. As you continue using the chaffle, it helps to suppress hunger and increase fat burning.

The chaffle is made with coconut and pumpkin, making it a healthy low-carb alternative for anyone looking to lose weight. When used as part of a healthy diet, the chaffle helps stabilize blood sugar levels so the body has an easier time sensing when food is needed. The keto chaffle contains no calories or carbs, making it an ideal tool for anyone looking to lose or maintain their weight.

Regularly, keto dieters' lookout for ways to be accurate on the diet while searching for ways to make life easier at that.

Chaffles are one of those foods that bring on a stimulating effect to the low-carb lifestyle. I find them to be an easy fix, and thankfully, they can be enjoyed different times of the day. In the recipes below, I share many ways to make and use chaffles —for breakfast through to dinner, snacks, and desserts.

This blend, therefore, makes dieting simpler as chaffles are enriched with healthy fats and mostly with no carbs. Reaching ketosis just got easier!

Finally, they are convenient for prep-ahead meals. And we know how prepping meals aids with effective keto dieting. Chaffles can be frozen for later use, and they taste excellent when warmed and enjoyed later.

Once you are hooked on chaffles, they will become a crucial part of your feeding because of the benefits that they bring. I have been making them continuously for weeks and thinking of creating a second cookbook of my new chaffle discoveries.

How to Make Chaffles?

Equipment and Ingredients Discussed

Making chaffles requires five simple steps and nothing more than a waffle maker for flat chaffles and a waffle bowl maker for chaffle bowls.

To make chaffles, you will need two necessary ingredients – eggs and cheese. My preferred cheeses are cheddar cheese or mozzarella cheese. These melt quickly, making them the go-to for most recipes. Meanwhile, always ensure that your cheeses are finely grated or thinly sliced for use.

Now, to make a standard chaffle:

- First, preheat your waffle maker until adequately hot.

- Meanwhile, in a bowl, mix the egg with cheese on hand until well combined.

- Open the iron, pour in a quarter or half of the mixture, and close.

- Cook the chaffle for 5 to 7 minutes or until it is crispy.

- Transfer the chaffle to a plate and allow cooling before serving.

11 Tips to Make Chaffles

My surefire ways to turn out the crispiest of chaffles:

- **Preheat Well:** Yes! It sounds obvious to preheat the waffle iron before usage. However, preheating the iron moderately will not get your chaffles as crispy as you will like. The best way to preheat before cooking is to ensure that the iron is very hot.

- **Not-So-Cheesy:** Will you prefer to have your chaffles less cheesy? Then, use mozzarella cheese.

- **Not-So Eggy**: If you aren't comfortable with the smell of eggs in your chaffles, try using egg whites instead of egg yolks or whole eggs.

- **To Shred or to Slice:** Many recipes call for shredded cheese when making chaffles, but I find sliced cheeses to offer crispier pieces. While I stick with mostly shredded cheese for convenience's sake, be at ease to use sliced cheese in the same quantity. When using sliced cheeses, arrange two to four pieces in the waffle iron, top with the beaten eggs, and some slices of the cheese. Cover and cook until crispy.

- **Shallower Irons:** For better crisps on your chaffles, use shallower waffle irons as they cook easier and faster.

- **Layering:** Don't fill up the waffle iron with too much batter. Work between a quarter and a half cup of total ingredients per batch for correctly done chaffles.

- **Patience:** It is a virtue even when making chaffles. For the best results, allow the chaffles to sit in the iron for 5 to 7 minutes before serving.

- **No Peeking:** 7 minutes isn't too much of a time to wait for the outcome of your chaffles, in my opinion. Opening the iron and checking on the chaffle before it is done stands you a worse chance of ruining it.

- **Crispy Cooling:** For better crisp, I find that allowing the chaffles to cool further after they are transferred to a plate aids a lot.

- **Easy Cleaning:** For the best cleanup, wet a paper towel and wipe the inner parts of the iron clean while still warm. Kindly note that the iron should be warm but not hot!

- **Brush It:** Also, use a clean toothbrush to clean between the iron's teeth for a thorough cleanup. You may also use a dry, rough sponge to clean the iron while it is still warm

SIMPLE CHAFFLES

1. Mayonnaise & Cream Cheese Chaffles

Preparation time: 9 minutes

Cooking Time: 20 Minutes

Servings: 2

Ingredients:

- 4 organic eggs large
- 4 tablespoons mayonnaise
- 1 tablespoon almond flour
- 2 tablespoons cream cheese, cut into small cubes

Directions:

1. Preheat a waffle iron and then grease it.
2. In a bowl, place the eggs, mayonnaise and almond flour and with a hand mixer, mix until smooth.
3. Place about ¼ of the mixture into preheated waffle iron.
4. Place about ¼ of the cream cheese cubes on top of the mixture evenly and cook for about 5 minutes or until golden brown.
5. Repeat with the remaining mixture and cream cheese cubes.

6. Serve warm.

Nutrition: Calories: 190Net Carb: 0.6gFat: 17gSaturated Fat: 4.2gCarbohydrates: 0.8gDietary Fiber: 0.2g Sugar: 0.5gProtein: 6.7g

2. Blue Cheese Chaffle Bites

Preparation time: 10 minutes

Cooking Time: 14 Minutes

Servings: 2

Ingredients:

- 1 egg, beaten
- ½ cup finely grated Parmesan cheese
- ¼ cup crumbled blue cheese
- 1 tsp erythritol

Directions:

1. Preheat the waffle iron.
2. Mix all the ingredients in a bowl.
3. Open the iron and add half of the mixture. Close and cook until crispy, 7 minutes.
4. Remove the chaffle onto a plate and make another with the remaining mixture.
5. Cut each chaffle into wedges and serve afterward.

Nutrition: Calories 19ats 13.91gCarbs 4.03gNet Carbs 4.03gProtein 13.48g

3. Raspberries Chaffles

Servings:2

Cooking Time: 5 Minutes

Ingredients:

- 1 egg
- 1/2 cup mozzarella cheese, shredded
- 1 tbsp. almond flour
- 1/4 cup raspberry puree
- 1 tbsp. coconut flour for topping

Directions:

1. Preheat your waffle maker in line with the manufacturer's instructions.
2. Grease your waffle maker with cooking spray.
3. Mix together egg, almond flour, and raspberry purée.
4. Add cheese and mix until well combined.
5. Pour batter into the waffle maker.
6. Close the lid.
7. Cook for about 3-4 minutes Utes or until waffles are cooked and not soggy.
8. Once cooked, remove from the maker.
9. Sprinkle coconut flour on top and enjoy!

Nutrition: Protein: 26% 60 kcal Fat: 63% 145 kcal Carbohydrates: 11% 25 kcal

4. Simple Chaffle Toast

Servings:2

Cooking Time: 5 Minutes

Ingredients:

- 1 large egg
- 1/2 cup shredded cheddar cheese
- FOR TOPPING
- 1 egg
- 3-4 spinach leaves
- ¼ cup boil and shredded chicken

Directions:

1. Preheat your square waffle maker on medium-high heat.
2. Mix together egg and cheese in a bowl and make two chaffles in a chaffle maker
3. Once chaffle are cooked, carefully remove them from the maker.
4. Serve with spinach, boiled chicken, and fried egg.
5. Serve hot and enjoy!

Nutrition: Protein: 39% 99 kcal Fat: % 153 kcal Carbohydrates: 1% 3 kcal

5. Savory Beef Chaffle

Preparation time: 10 minutes

Cooking Time: 15 Minutes

Servings: 2

Ingredients:

- 1 teaspoon olive oil
- 2 cups ground beef
- Garlic salt to taste
- 1 red bell pepper, sliced into strips
- 1 green bell pepper, sliced into strips
- 1 onion, minced
- 1 bay leaf
- 2 garlic chaffles
- Butter

Directions:

1. Put your pan over medium heat.
2. Add the olive oil and cook ground beef until brown.
3. Season with garlic salt and add bay leaf.
4. Drain the fat, transfer to a plate and set aside.
5. Discard the bay leaf.

6. In the same pan, cook the onion and bell peppers for 2 minutes.

7. Put the beef back to the pan.

8. Heat for 1 minute.

9. Spread butter on top of the chaffle.

10. Add the ground beef and veggies.

11. Roll or fold the chaffle.

Nutrition: Calories 220 Total Fat 17.8g Saturated Fat 8g Cholesterol 76mg Sodium 60mg Total Carbohydrate 3g Dietary Fiber 2g Total Sugars 5.4g Protein 27.1g Potassium 537mg

6. Chaffles With Almond Flour

Servings:4

Cooking Time: 5 Minutes

Ingredients:

- 2 large eggs
- 1/4 cup almond flour
- 3/4 tsp baking powder
- 1 cup cheddar cheese, shredded
- Cooking spray

Directions:

1. Switch on your waffle maker and grease with cooking spray.
2. Beat eggs with almond flour and baking powder in a mixing bowl.
3. Once the eggs and cheese are mixed together, add in cheese and mix again.
4. Pour 1/cup of the batter in the dash mini waffle maker and close the lid.
5. Cook chaffles for about 2-3 minutes until crispy and cooked
6. Repeat with the remaining batter
7. Carefully transfer the chaffles to plate.

8. Serve with almonds and enjoy!

Nutrition: Protein: 23% 52 kcal Fat: 72% 15kcal Carbohydrates: 5% 11 kcal

7. Nutter Butter Chaffles

Preparation time: 10 minutes

Cooking Time: 14 Minutes

Servings: 2

Ingredients:

- For the chaffles:
- 2 tbsp sugar-free peanut butter powder
- 2 tbsp maple (sugar-free) syrup
- 1 egg, beaten
- ¼ cup finely grated mozzarella cheese
- ¼ tsp baking powder
- ¼ tsp almond butter
- ¼ tsp peanut butter extract
- 1 tbsp softened cream cheese
- For the frosting:
- ½ cup almond flour
- 1 cup peanut butter
- 3 tbsp almond milk
- ½ tsp vanilla extract
- ½ cup maple (sugar-free) syrup

Directions:

1. Preheat the waffle iron.

2. Meanwhile, in a medium bowl, mix all the ingredients until smooth.

3. Open the iron and pour in half of the mixture.

4. Close the iron and cook until crispy, 6 to 7 minutes.

5. Remove the chaffle onto a plate and set aside.

6. Make a second chaffle with the remaining batter.

7. While the chaffles cool, make the frosting.

8. Pour the almond flour in a medium saucepan and stir-fry over medium heat until golden.

9. Transfer the almond flour to a blender and top with the remaining frosting ingredients. Process until smooth.

10. Spread the frosting on the chaffles and serve afterward.

Nutrition: Calories 239Fats 15.48gCarbs 17.42gNet Carbs 15.92gProtein 7.52g

8. Keto Reuben Chaffles

Preparation time: 9 minutes

Cooking Time: 28 Minutes

Servings: 2

Ingredients:

- For the chaffles:
- 2 eggs, beaten
- 1 cup finely grated Swiss cheese
- 2 tsp caraway seeds
- 1/8 tsp salt
- ½ tsp baking powder
- For the sauce:
- 2 tbsp sugar-free ketchup
- 3 tbsp mayonnaise
- 1 tbsp dill relish
- 1 tsp hot sauce
- For the filling:
- 6 oz pastrami
- 2 Swiss cheese slices
- ¼ cup pickled radishes

Directions:

1. For the chaffles:
2. Preheat the waffle iron.
3. In a medium bowl, mix the eggs, Swiss cheese, caraway seeds, salt, and baking powder.
4. Open the iron and add a quarter of the mixture. Close and cook until crispy, 7 minutes.
5. Transfer the chaffle to a plate and make 3 more chaffles in the same manner.
6. For the sauce:
7. In another bowl, mix the ketchup, mayonnaise, dill relish, and hot sauce.
8. To assemble:
9. Divide on two chaffles; the sauce, the pastrami, Swiss cheese slices, and pickled radishes.
10. Cover with the other chaffles, divide the sandwich in halves and serve.

Nutrition: Calories 316Fats 21.78gCarbs 6.52gNet Carbs 5.42gProtein 23.56g

9. Carrot Chaffle Cake

Servings: 6

Cooking Time: 24 Minutes

Ingredients:

- 1 egg, beaten
- 2 tablespoons melted butter
- ½ cup carrot, shredded
- ¾ cup almond flour
- 1 teaspoon baking powder
- 2 tablespoons heavy whipping cream
- 2 tablespoons sweetener
- 1 tablespoon walnuts, chopped
- 1 teaspoon pumpkin spice
- 2 teaspoons cinnamon

Directions:

1. Preheat your waffle maker.
2. In a large bowl, combine all the ingredients.
3. Pour some of the mixture into the waffle maker.
4. Close and cook for minutes.

5. Repeat steps until all the remaining batter has been used.

Nutrition: Calories   294Total   Fat   27g Saturated   Fat 12g Cholesterol   133mg Sodium   144mg Potassium 421mgTotal Carbohydrate 11.6g Dietary Fiber 4.5g Protein 6.8g Total Sugars 1.7g

10. Colby Jack Slices Chaffles

Preparation time: 8 minutes

Cooking Time: 6 Minutes

Servings: 2

Ingredients:

- 2 ounces Colby Jack cheese, cut into thin triangle slices
- 1 large organic egg, beaten

Directions:

1. Preheat a waffle iron and then grease it.
2. Arrange 1 thin layer of cheese slices in the bottom of preheated waffle iron.
3. Place the beaten egg on top of the cheese.
4. Now, arrange another layer of cheese slices on top to cover evenly.
5. Cook for about 6 minutes or until golden brown.
6. Serve warm.

Nutrition: Calories: 292Net Carb: 2.4gFat: 23gSaturated Fat: 13.6gCarbohydrates: 2.4gDietary Fiber: 0g Sugar: 0.4gProtein: 18.3g

BREAKFAST CHAFFLE RECIPE

11. Crispy Chaffles With Egg & Asparagus

Preparation Time: 10 minutes

Servings:1

Cooking Time: 10 Minutes

Ingredients:

- 1 egg
- 1/4 cup cheddar cheese
- 2 tbsps. almond flour
- ½ tsp. baking powder
- TOPPING
- 1 egg
- 4-5 stalks asparagus
- 1 tsp avocado oil

Directions:

1. Preheat waffle maker to medium-high heat.
2. Whisk together egg, mozzarella cheese, almond flour, and baking powder

3. Pour chaffles mixture into the center of the waffle iron. Close the waffle maker and let cook for 5 minutes Utes or until waffle is golden brown and set.

4. Remove chaffles from the waffle maker and serve.

5. Meanwhile, heat oil in a nonstick pan.

6. Once the pan is hot, fry asparagus for about 4-5 minutes Utes until golden brown.

7. Poach the egg in boil water for about 2-3 minutes Utes.

8. Once chaffles are cooked, remove from the maker.

9. Serve chaffles with the poached egg and asparagus.

Nutrition: Protein: 26% 85 kcal Fat: 69% 226 kcal Carbohydrates: 5% 16 kcal

12. Delicious Raspberries taco Chaffles

Preparation Time: 10 minutes

Servings:1

Cooking Time: 15 Minutes

Ingredients:

- 1 egg white
- 1/4 cup jack cheese, shredded
- 1/4 cup cheddar cheese, shredded
- 1 tsp coconut flour
- 1/4 tsp baking powder
- 1/2 tsp stevia
- For Topping
- 4 oz. raspberries
- 2 tbsps. coconut flour
- 2 oz. unsweetened raspberry sauce

Directions:

1. Switch on your round Waffle Maker and grease it with cooking spray once it is hot.

2. Mix together all chaffle ingredients in a bowl and combine with a fork.

3. Pour chaffle batter in a preheated maker and close the lid.

4. Roll the taco chaffle around using a kitchen roller, set it aside and allow it to set for a few minutes Utes.

5. Once the taco chaffle is set, remove from the roller.

6. Dip raspberries in sauce and arrange on taco chaffle.

7. Drizzle coconut flour on top.

8. Enjoy raspberries taco chaffle with keto coffee.

Nutrition: Protein: 28% 77 kcal Fat: 6 187 kcal Carbohydrates: 3% 8 kcal

13. __Coconut Chaffles__

Preparation Time: 10 minutes

Servings:2

Cooking Time: 5 Minutes

Ingredients:

- 1 egg
- 1 oz. cream cheese,
- 1 oz. cheddar cheese
- 2 tbsps. coconut flour
- 1 tsp. stevia
- 1 tbsp. coconut oil, melted
- 1/2 tsp. coconut extract
- 2 eggs, soft boil for serving

Directions:

1. Heat you minutes Dash waffle maker and grease with cooking spray.
2. Mix together all chaffles ingredients in a bowl.
3. Pour chaffle batter in a preheated waffle maker.
4. Close the lid.
5. Cook chaffles for about 2-3 minutes Utes until golden brown.

6. Serve with boil egg and enjoy!

Nutrition: Protein: 21% 32 kcal Fat: % 117 kcal Carbohydrates: 3% 4 kcal

14. Garlic and Parsley Chaffles

Preparation Time: 10 minutes

Servings:1

Cooking Time: 5 Minutes

Ingredients:

- 1 large egg
- 1/4 cup cheese mozzarella
- 1 tsp. coconut flour
- ¼ tsp. baking powder
- ½ tsp. garlic powder
- 1 tbsp. minutes parsley
- For Serving
- 1 Poach egg
- 4 oz. smoked salmon

Directions:

1. Switch on your Dash minutes waffle maker and let it preheat.
2. Grease waffle maker with cooking spray.
3. Mix together egg, mozzarella, coconut flour, baking powder, and garlic powder, parsley to a mixing bowl until combined well.

4. Pour batter in circle chaffle maker.

5. Close the lid.

6. Cook for about 2-3 minutes Utes or until the chaffles are cooked.

7. Serve with smoked salmon and poached egg.

8. Enjoy!

Nutrition: Protein: 45% 140 kcal Fat: 51% 160 kcal Carbohydrates: 4% 14 kcal

15. Scrambled Eggs on A Spring Onion Chaffle

Preparation Time: 10 minutes

Servings:4

Cooking Time:7–9 Minutes

Ingredients:

- Batter
- 4 eggs
- 2 cups grated mozzarella cheese
- 2 spring onions, finely chopped
- Salt and pepper to taste
- ½ teaspoon dried garlic powder
- 2 tablespoons almond flour
- 2 tablespoons coconut flour
- Other
- 2 tablespoons butter for brushing the waffle maker
- 6-8 eggs
- Salt and pepper
- 1 teaspoon Italian spice mix
- 1 tablespoon olive oil
- 1 tablespoon freshly chopped parsley

Directions:

1. Preheat the waffle maker.

2. Crack the eggs into a bowl and add the grated cheese.

3. Mix until just combined, then add the chopped spring onions and season with salt and pepper and dried garlic powder.

4. Stir in the almond flour and mix until everything is combined.

5. Brush the heated waffle maker with butter and add a few tablespoons of the batter.

6. Close the lid and cook for about 7–8 minutes depending on your waffle maker.

7. While the chaffles are cooking, prepare the scrambled eggs by whisking the eggs in a bowl until frothy, about 2 minutes. Season with salt and black pepper to taste and add the Italian spice mix. Whisk to blend in the spices.

8. Warm the oil in a non-stick pan over medium heat.

9. Pour the eggs in the pan and cook until eggs are set to your liking.

10. Serve each chaffle and top with some scrambled eggs. Top with freshly chopped parsley.

Nutrition: Calories 194, fat 14.7 g, carbs 5 g, sugar 0.6 g, Protein 1 g, sodium 191 mg

16. Egg on A Cheddar Cheese Chaffle

Preparation Time: 10 minutes

Servings:4

Cooking Time:7–9 Minutes

Ingredients:

- Batter
- 4 eggs
- 2 cups shredded white cheddar cheese
- Salt and pepper to taste
- Other
- 2 tablespoons butter for brushing the waffle maker
- 4 large eggs
- 2 tablespoons olive oil

Directions:

1. Preheat the waffle maker.
2. Crack the eggs into a bowl and whisk them with a fork.
3. Stir in the grated cheddar cheese and season with salt and pepper.
4. Brush the heated waffle maker with butter and add a few tablespoons of the batter.

5. Close the lid and cook for about 7–8 minutes depending on your waffle maker.

6. While chaffles are cooking, cook the eggs.

7. Warm the oil in a large non-stick pan that has a lid over medium-low heat for 2-3 minutes

8. Crack an egg in a small ramekin and gently add it to the pan. Repeat the same way for the other 3 eggs.

9. Cover and let cook for 2 to 2 ½ minutes for set eggs but with runny yolks.

10. Remove from heat.

11. To serve, place a chaffle on each plate and top with an egg. Season with salt and black pepper to taste.

Nutrition: Calories 4 fat 34 g, carbs 2 g, sugar 0.6 g, Protein 26 g, sodium 518 mg

17. Avocado Chaffle Toast

Preparation Time: 10 minutes

Servings:3

Cooking Time: 10 Minutes

Ingredients:

- 4 tbsps. avocado mash
- 1/2 tsp lemon juice
- 1/8 tsp salt
- 1/8 tsp black pepper
- 2 eggs
- 1/2 cup shredded cheese
- For serving
- 3 eggs
- ½ avocado thinly sliced
- 1 tomato, sliced

Directions:

1. Mash avocado mash with lemon juice, salt, and black pepper in mixing bowl, until well combined.
2. In a small bowl beat egg and pour eggs in avocado mixture and mix well.
3. Switch on Waffle Maker to pre-heat.

4. Pour 1/8 of shredded cheese in a waffle maker and then pour ½ of egg and avocado mixture and then 1/8 shredded cheese.

5. Close the lid and cook chaffles for about 3 - 4 minutes Utes.

6. Repeat with the remaining mixture.

7. Meanwhile, fry eggs in a pan for about 1-2 minutes Utes.

8. For serving, arrange fried egg on chaffle toast with avocado slice and tomatoes.

9. Sprinkle salt and pepper on top and enjoy!

Nutrition: Protein: 26% 66 kcal Fat: 67% 169 kcal Carbohydrates: 6% 15 kcal

18. Cajun & Feeta Chaffles

Preparation Time: 10 minutes

Servings:1

Cooking Time: 10 Minutes

Ingredients:

- 1 egg white
- 1/4 cup shredded mozzarella cheese
- 2 tbsps. almond flour
- 1 tsp Cajun Seasoning
- FOR SERVING
- 1 egg
- 4 oz. feta cheese
- 1 tomato, sliced

Directions:

1. Whisk together egg, cheese, and seasoning in a bowl.
2. Switch on and grease waffle maker with cooking spray.
3. Pour batter in a preheated waffle maker.
4. Cook chaffles for about 2-3 minutes Utes until the chaffle is cooked through.
5. Meanwhile, fry the egg in a non-stick pan for about 1-2 minutes Utes.

6. For serving set fried egg on chaffles with feta cheese and tomatoes slice.

Nutrition: Protein: 28% 119 kcal Fat: 64% 2 kcal Carbohydrates: 7% 31 kcal

19. Crispy Chaffles With Sausage

Preparation Time: 10 minutes

Servings:2

Cooking Time: 10 Minutes

Ingredients:

- 1/2 cup cheddar cheese
- 1/2 tsp. baking powder
- 1/4 cup egg whites
- 2 tsp. pumpkin spice
- 1 egg, whole
- 2 chicken sausage
- 2 slice bacon
- salt and pepper to taste
- 1 tsp. avocado oil

Directions:

1. Mix together all ingredients in a bowl.
2. Allow batter to sit while waffle iron warms.
3. Spray waffle iron with nonstick spray.
4. Pour batter in the waffle maker and cook according to the directions of the manufacturer.

5. Meanwhile, heat oil in a pan and fry the egg, according to your choice and transfer it to plate.

6. In the same pan, fry bacon slice and sausage on medium heat for about 2-3 minutes Utes until cooked.

7. Once chaffles are cooked thoroughly, remove them from the maker.

8. Serve with fried egg, bacon slice, sausages and enjoy!

Nutrition: Protein: 22% 86 kcal Fat: 74% 286 kcal Carbohydrates: 3% 12 kcal

20. Chili Chaffle

Preparation Time: 10 minutes

Servings:4

Cooking Time:7–9 Minutes

Ingredients:

- Batter
- 4 eggs
- ½ cup grated parmesan cheese
- 1½ cups grated yellow cheddar cheese
- 1 hot red chili pepper
- Salt and pepper to taste
- ½ teaspoon dried garlic powder
- 1 teaspoon dried basil
- 2 tablespoons almond flour
- Other
- 2 tablespoons olive oil for brushing the waffle maker

Directions:

1. Preheat the waffle maker.
2. Crack the eggs into a bowl and add the grated parmesan and cheddar cheese.

3. Mix until just combined and add the chopped chili pepper. Season with salt and pepper, dried garlic powder and dried basil. Stir in the almond flour.

4. Mix until everything is combined.

5. Brush the heated waffle maker with olive oil and add a few tablespoons of the batter.

6. Close the lid and cook for about 7–8 minutes depending on your waffle maker.

Nutrition: Calories 36 fat 30.4 g, carbs 3.1 g, sugar 0.7 g, Protein 21.5 g, sodium 469 mg

BASIC CHAFFLES

21. White Bread Keto Chaffle

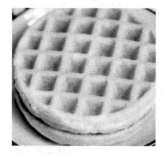

Preparation time: 5 minutes

Cooking time: 4 minutes

Servings: 2

Ingredients

- 2 egg whites
- cream cheese, melted
- 2 tsp water
- 1/4 tsp baking powder
- 1/4 cup almond flour
- 1 Pinch of salt

Directions

1. Pre-heat the mini waffle maker,

2. Whisk the egg whites together with the cream cheese and water in a bowl.

3. Next step is to add the baking powder, almond flour and salt and whisk until you have a smooth batter. Then you pour half of the batter into the mini waffle maker.

4. Allow to cook for roughly 4 minutes or until you no longer see steam coming from the waffle maker.

5. Remove and allow to cool.

Nutrition: Calories 320 Carbohydrates 2.9 g Protein 21.5 g Fat 24.3g

22. Cranberry and Brie Chaffle

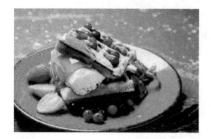

Preparation time: 10 minutes

Cooking time: 20 minutes

Servings: 4 mini chaffles

Ingredients:

- 4 tablespoons frozen cranberries

- 3 tablespoons swerve sweetener

- 1 cup / 115 grams shredded brie cheese

- 2 eggs, at room temperature

Directions:

1. Take a non-stick waffle iron, plug it in, select the medium or medium-high heat setting and let it preheat until ready to use; it could also be indicated with an indicator light changing its color.

2. Meanwhile, prepare the batter and for this, take a heatproof bowl, add cheese in it, and microwave at

high heat setting for 15 seconds or until cheese has softened.

3. Then add sweetener, berries, and egg into the cheese and whisk with an electric mixer until smooth.

4. Use a ladle to pour one-fourth of the prepared batter into the heated waffle iron in a spiral direction, starting from the edges, then shut the lid and cook for 4 minutes or more until solid and nicely browned; the cooked waffle will look like a cake.

5. When done, transfer chaffles to a plate with a silicone spatula and repeat with the remaining batter.

6. Let chaffles stand for some time until crispy and serve straight away.

Nutrition: Calories 320 Carbohydrates 2.9 g Protein 21.5 g Fat 24.3g

23. Banana Foster Chaffle

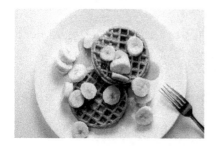

Preparation time: 10 minutes

Cooking time: 20 minutes

Servings: 4 large chaffles

Ingredients:

- For Chaffle:
- 1/8 teaspoon cinnamon
- ½ teaspoon banana extract, unsweetened
- 4 teaspoons swerve sweetener
- 1 cup / 225 grams cream cheese, softened
- ½ teaspoon vanilla extract, unsweetened
- 8 eggs, at room temperature
- For Syrup:
- 20 drops of banana extract, unsweetened
- 8 teaspoons swerve sweetener
- 20 drops of caramel extract, unsweetened
- 12 drops of rum extract, unsweetened

- 8 tablespoons unsalted butter

- 1/8 teaspoon cinnamon

Directions:

1. Take a non-stick waffle iron, plug it in, select the medium or medium-high heat setting and let it preheat until ready to use; it could also be indicated with an indicator light changing its color.

2. Meanwhile, prepare the batter for chaffle and for this, take a large bowl, crack eggs in it, add sweetener, cream cheese, and all the extracts and then mix with an electric mixer until smooth, let the batter stand for 5 minutes.

3. Use a ladle to pour one-fourth of the prepared batter into the heated waffle iron in a spiral direction, starting from the edges, then shut the lid and cook for 5 minutes or more until solid and nicely browned; the cooked waffle will look like a cake.

4. When done, transfer chaffles to a plate with a silicone spatula, repeat with the remaining batter and let chaffles stand for some time until crispy.

5. Meanwhile, prepare the syrup and for this, take a small heatproof bowl, add butter in it, and microwave at high heat setting for 15 seconds until it melts.

6. Then add remaining ingredients for the syrup and mix until combined.

7. Drizzle syrup over chaffles and then serve.

Nutrition: Calories 320 Carbohydrates 2.9 g Protein 21.5 g Fat 24.3g

24. **Flaxseed Chaffle**

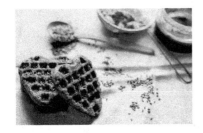

Preparation time: 10 minutes

Cooking time: 20 minutes

Servings: 4 medium chaffles

Ingredients:

- 2 cups ground flaxseed

- 2 teaspoons ground cinnamon

- 1 teaspoon of sea salt

- 1 tablespoon baking powder

- 1/3 cup / 80 ml avocado oil

- 5 eggs, at room temperature

- ½ cup / 120 ml water

- Whipped cream as needed for topping

Directions:

1. Take a non-stick waffle iron, plug it in, select the medium or medium-high heat setting and let it preheat

until ready to use; it could also be indicated with an indicator light changing its color.

2. Meanwhile, prepare the batter and for this, take a large bowl and then stir in flaxseed, salt and baking powder until combined.

3. Crack the eggs in a jug, pour in oil and water, whisk these ingredients until blended and then stir this mixture into the flour with the spatula until incorporated and fluffy mixture comes together.

4. Let the batter stand for 5 minutes and then stir in cinnamon until mixed.

5. Use a ladle to pour one-fourth of the prepared batter into the heated waffle iron in a spiral direction, starting from the edges, then shut the lid and cook for 5 minutes or more until solid and nicely browned; the cooked waffle will look like a cake.

6. When done, transfer chaffle to a plate with a silicone spatula and repeat with the remaining batter.

7. Top waffles with whipped cream and then serve straight away.

Nutrition: Calories 320 Carbohydrates 2.9 g Protein 21.5 g Fat 24.3g

25. Hazelnut Chaffle

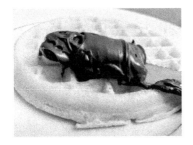

Preparation time: 10 minutes

Cooking time: 30 minutes

Servings: 6 mini chaffles

Ingredients:

- 1 cup / 100 grams hazelnut flour
- ½ teaspoon baking powder
- 2 tablespoons hazelnut oil
- 1 cup / 245 grams almond milk, unsweetened
- 3 eggs, at room temperature

Directions:

1. Take a non-stick waffle iron, plug it in, select the medium or medium-high heat setting and let it preheat until ready to use; it could also be indicated with an indicator light changing its color.

2. Meanwhile, prepare the batter and for this, take a large bowl, add flour in it, stir in the baking powder until

mixed and then mix in oil, milk, and egg with an electric mixer until smooth.

3. Use a ladle to pour one-sixth of the prepared batter into the heated waffle iron in a spiral direction, starting from the edges, then shut the lid and cook for 5 minutes or more until solid and nicely browned; the cooked waffle will look like a cake.

4. When done, transfer chaffle to a plate with a silicone spatula and repeat with the remaining batter.

5. Let chaffles stand for some time until crispy and serve straight away.

Nutrition: Calories 320 Carbohydrates 2.9 g Protein 21.5 g Fat 24.3g

26. Maple Pumpkin Chaffle

Preparation time: 5 minutes

Cooking time: 4 minutes

Servings: 2

Ingredients:

- 2 eggs
- 3/4 tsp baking powder
- 2 tsp 100% pumpkin puree
- 3/4 tsp pumpkin pie spice
- 4 tsp heavy whipping cream
- 2 tsp sugar-free maple syrup
- 1 tsp coconut flour
- 1/2 cup mozzarella cheese, shredded
- 1/2 tsp vanilla
- Pinch of salt

Directions:

1. Preheat the waffle maker.
2. Combine all ingredients in a small mixing bowl.
3. If you're using a mini waffle maker, pour around 1/4 of the batter. Allow to cook for 3-4 minutes.
4. Repeat.

Nutrition: Calories 320 Carbohydrates 2.9 g Protein 21.5 g Fat 24.3g

27. <u>Nutty Chaffles</u>

Preparation time: 5 minutes

Cooking time: 5 minutes

Servings: 1

Ingredients:

- 1 egg
- 1 tsp coconut flour
- 1 1/2 tbsp unsweetened cocoa
- 2 tbsp sugar-free sweetener
- 1 tbsp heavy cream
- 1/2 tsp baking powder
- 1/2 tsp vanilla

Directions:

1. Preheat the waffle maker.
2. Combine all the ingredients in a small bowl. Mix well.
3. Pour half the batter into the waffle maker. Allow to cook for 3-5 minutes until golden brown and crispy.
4. Carefully remove and add the remaining batter.

Nutrition: Calories 320 Carbohydrates 2.9 g Protein 21.5 g Fat 24.3g

28. Crispy Chaffle With Everything but The Bagel Seasoning

Preparation time: 5 minutes

Cooking time: 5 minutes

Servings: 1

Ingredients:

- 2 eggs
- 1/2 cup parmesan cheese
- 1 tsp everything but the bagel seasoning
- 1/2 cup mozzarella cheese
- 2 tsp almond flour

Directions:

1. Preheat the waffle maker.
2. Sprinkle the mozzarella cheese onto the waffle maker. Let it melt and cook for 30 seconds until crispy. Remove this from the waffle maker.
3. Using a whisk, combine eggs, parmesan, almond flour, seasoning, and the toasted cheese in a small bowl.
4. Pour the batter into the waffle maker.
5. Allow the batter to cook for 3-4 minutes until crispy and golden brown in color.

Nutrition: Calories 320 Carbohydrates 2.9 g Protein 21.5 g Fat 24.3g

29. Strawberry and Cream Cheese Low-Carb Keto Waffles

Preparation time: 5 minutes

Cooking time: 5 minutes

Servings: 2

Ingredients:

- 2 tsp coconut flour
- 4 tsp monk fruit
- 1/4 tsp baking powder
- 1 egg
- 1 oz cream cheese, softened
- 1/2 tsp vanilla extract
- 1/4 cup strawberries

Directions:

1. Preheat the waffle maker.
2. In a bowl put in the coconut flour, then add the baking powder and the monk fruit.
3. Add in the egg, cream cheese, and vanilla extract. Mix well with a whisk.
4. Pour the batter into the preheated waffle maker and allow to cook for 3-4 minutes.

5. Allow chaffles to cool before topping with strawberries.

Nutrition: Calories 320 Carbohydrates 2.9 g Protein 21.5 g Fat 24.3g

30. Pumpkin Chaffle With Cream Cheese Glaze

Preparation time: 5 minutes

Cooking time: 5 minutes

Servings: 1

Ingredients:

- 1 egg
- 1/2 cup mozzarella cheese
- 1/2 tsp pumpkin pie spice
- 1 tbsp pumpkin
- For the cream cheese frosting:
- 2 tbsp cream cheese, softened at room temperature
- 2 tbsp monk fruit
- 1/2 tsp vanilla extract

Directions:

1. Preheat the waffle maker.
2. Whip the egg in a small bowl.
3. Add cheese, pumpkin, and pumpkin pie spice to the whipped egg and mix well.
4. Add half the batter to the waffle maker and allow to cook for 3-4 minutes.

5. While waiting for the chaffle to cook, combine all the ingredients for the frosting in another bowl. Continue mixing until a smooth and creamy consistency is reached. Feel free to add more butter if you prefer a buttery taste.

Nutrition: Calories 320 Carbohydrates 2.9 g Protein 21.5 g Fat 24.3g

Allow the chaffle to cool before frosting it with cream cheese.

31. Crunch Cereal Cake Chaffle

Preparation time: 10 minutes

Cooking time: 5 minutes

Servings: 1

(Does not include the toppings)

Ingredients:

- For the chaffles:
- 1 egg
- 2 tbsp almond flour
- 1/2 tsp coconut flour
- 1 tbsp butter, melted
- 1 tbsp cream cheese, softened
- 1/4 tsp vanilla extract
- 1/4 tsp baking powder
- 1 tbsp confectioners' sweetener
- 1/8 tsp xanthan gum
- For the toppings:
- 20 drops captain cereal flavoring
- Whipped cream

Directions:

1. Preheat the mini waffle maker.

2. Blend or mix all the chaffles ingredients until the consistency is creamy and smooth. Allow to rest for a few minutes so that the flour absorbs the liquid ingredients.
3. Scoop out 2-3 tbsp of batter and put it into the waffle maker. Allow to cook for 2-3 minutes.
4. Top the cooked chaffles with freshly whipped cream.
5. Add syrup and drops of Captain Cereal flavoring for a great flavor.

Nutrition: Calories 120 Carbohydrates 1.9 g Protein 21.5 g Fat 24.3g

SWEET CHAFFLES

32. Spiced Pumpkin Chaffles

Preparation time: 5 minutes

Cooking Time: 8 Minutes

Servings: 2

Ingredients:

- 1 organic egg, beaten
- ½ cup Mozzarella cheese, shredded
- 1 tablespoon sugar-free canned solid pumpkin
- ¼ teaspoon ground cinnamon
- Pinch of ground cloves
- Pinch of ground nutmeg
- Pinch of ground ginger

Directions:

1. Preheat a mini waffle iron and then grease it.
2. In a medium bowl, place all ingredients and with a fork, mix until well combined.
3. Place half of the mixture into preheated waffle iron and cook for about 4 minutes or until golden brown.

4. Repeat with the remaining mixture.

5. Serve warm.

Nutrition: Calories: 5et Carb: 1gFat: 3.5gSaturated Fat: 1.5gCarbohydrates: 1.4gDietary Fiber: 0.4g Sugar: 0.5gProtein: 4.9g

33. Vanilla Chaffle

Preparation time: 5 minutes

Cooking Time: 8 Minutes

Servings: 4

Ingredients:

- 2 tbsp butter, softened
- 2 oz cream cheese, softened
- 2 eggs
- ¼ cup almond flour
- 2 tbsp coconut flour
- 1 tsp baking powder
- 1 tsp vanilla extract
- ¼ cup confectioners
- Pinch of pink salt

Directions:

1. Preheat the waffle maker and spray with non-stick cooking spray.
2. Melt the butter and set aside for a minute to cool.
3. Add the eggs into the melted butter and whisk until creamy.

4. Pour in the sweetener, vanilla, extract, and salt. Blend properly.

5. Next add the coconut flour, almond flour, and baking powder. Mix well.

6. Pour into the waffle maker and cook for 4 minutes.

7. Repeat the process with the remaining batter.

8. Remove and set aside to cool.

9. Enjoy.

Nutrition: Calories per Preparation time: 5 minutes 02 Kcal

; Fats: 27 g ; Carbs: 9 g ; Protein: 23 g

34. **Banana Nut Chaffle**

Preparation time: 5 minutes

Servings: 1

Cooking Time: 10 Minutes

Ingredients:

- 1 egg
- 1 Tbsp cream cheese, softened and room temp
- 1 Tbsp sugar-free cheesecake pudding
- ½ cup mozzarella cheese
- 1 Tbsp monk fruit confectioners' sweetener
- ¼ tsp vanilla extract
- ¼ tsp banana extract
- toppings of choice

Directions:

1. Turn on waffle maker to heat and oil it with cooking spray.
2. Beat egg in a small bowl.
3. Add remaining ingredients and mix until well incorporated.
4. Add one half of the batter to waffle maker and cook for minutes, until golden brown.

5. Remove chaffle and add the other half of the batter.

6. Top with your optional toppings and serve warm!

Nutrition: Carbs: 2 g ;Fat: g ;Protein: 8 g ;Calories: 119

35. Chocolaty Chips Pumpkin Chaffles

Preparation time: 5 minutes

Servings: 3

Cooking Time: 12 Minutes

Ingredients:

- 1 organic egg
- 4 teaspoons homemade pumpkin puree
- ½ cup Mozzarella cheese, shredded
- 1 tablespoon almond flour
- 2 tablespoons granulated Erythritol
- ¼ teaspoon pumpkin pie spice
- 4 teaspoons 70% dark chocolate chips

Directions:

1. In a bowl, place the egg and pumpkin puree and mix well.
2. Add the remaining ingredients except for chocolate chips and mix until well combined.
3. Gently, fold in the chocolate chips and lemon zest.
4. Place 1/3 of the mixture into preheated waffle iron and cook for about minutes or until golden brown.
5. Repeat with the remaining mixture.

6. Serve warm.

Nutrition: Calories: 9et Carb: 1.9gFat: 7.1gSaturated Fat: 3.3gCarbohydrates: 1.4gDietary Fiber: 2.6g Sugar: 0.4gProtein: 4.2g

36. Oreo Chaffles

Preparation time: 5 minutes

Cooking Time: 5 Minutes

Servings: 3

Ingredients:

- Chocolate Chaffle:
- 2 eggs
- 2 tbsp cocoa, unsweetened
- 2 tbsp sweetener
- 2 tbsp heavy cream
- 2 tsp coconut flour
- 1/2 tsp baking powder
- 1 tsp vanilla
- Filling:
- Whipped cream

Directions:

1. Pour half of the mixture into the waffle iron. Cook for 5 minutes.
2. Once ready, carefully remove and repeat with the remaining chaffle mixture.
3. Allow the cooked chaffles to sit for 3 minutes.

4. Once they have cooled, spread the whipped cream on the chaffles and stack them cream side facing down to form a sandwich.

5. Slice into halves and enjoy.

Nutrition: Calories per Servings: 390 Kcal ; Fats: 40 g ;

Carbs: 3 g ; Protein: 10 g

37. Whipping Cream Pumpkin Chaffles

Preparation time: 8 minutes

Cooking Time: 12 Minutes

Servings: 2

Ingredients:

- 2 organic eggs
- 2 tablespoons homemade pumpkin puree
- 2 tablespoons heavy whipping cream
- 1 tablespoon coconut flour
- 1 tablespoon Erythritol
- 1 teaspoon pumpkin pie spice
- ½ teaspoon organic baking powder
- ½ teaspoon organic vanilla extract
- Pinch of salt
- ½ cup Mozzarella cheese, shredded

Directions:

1. Preheat a mini waffle iron and then grease it.
2. In a bowl, place all the ingredients except Mozzarella cheese and beat until well combined.
3. Add the Mozzarella cheese and stir to combine.

4. Place half of the mixture into preheated waffle iron and cook for about 6 minutes or until golden brown.

5. Repeat with the remaining mixture.

6. Serve warm.

Nutrition: Calories: 81Net Carb: 2.1gFat: 5.9gSaturated Fat: 3gCarbohydrates: 3.1gDietary Fiber: 1g Sugar: 0.5gProtein: 4.3g

38. Chocolate Vanilla Chaffles

Preparation time: 5 minutes

Cooking Time: 5 Minutes

Servings: 2

Ingredients:

- ½ cup shredded mozzarella cheese
- 1 egg
- 1 Tbsp granulated sweetener
- 1 tsp vanilla extract
- 1 Tbsp sugar-free chocolate chips
- 2 Tbsp almond meal/flour

Directions:

1. Turn on waffle maker to heat and oil it with cooking spray.
2. Mix all components in a bowl until combined.
3. Pour half of the batter into waffle maker.
4. Cook for 2-minutes, then remove and repeat with remaining batter.
5. Top with more chips and favorite toppings.

Nutrition: Carbs: 23 g ;Fat: 3 g ;Protein: 4 g ;Calories: 134

39. Churro Waffles

Preparation time: 5 minutes

Servings: 1

Cooking Time: 10 Minutes

Ingredients:

- 1 tbsp coconut cream
- 1 egg
- 6 tbsp almond flour
- ¼ tsp xanthan gum
- ½ tsp cinnamon
- 2 tbsp keto brown sugar
- Coating:
- 2 tbsp butter, melt
- 1 tbsp keto brown sugar
- Warm up your waffle maker.

Directions:

1. Pour half of the batter to the waffle pan and cook for 5 minutes.
2. Carefully remove the cooked waffle and repeat the steps with the remaining batter.

3. Allow the chaffles to cool and spread with the melted butter and top with the brown sugar.

4. Enjoy.

Nutrition: Calories per Servings: 178 Kcal ; Fats: 15.7 g ;

Carbs: 3.9 g ; Protein: 2 g

40. Chocolate Chips Lemon Chaffles

Preparation time: 8 minutes

Cooking Time: 8 Minutes

Servings: 2

Ingredients:

- 2 organic eggs
- ½ cup Mozzarella cheese, shredded
- ¾ teaspoon organic lemon extract
- ½ teaspoon organic vanilla extract
- 2 teaspoons Erythritol
- ½ teaspoon psyllium husk powder
- Pinch of salt
- 1 tablespoon 70% dark chocolate chips
- ¼ teaspoon lemon zest, grated finely

Directions:

1. Preheat a mini waffle iron and then grease it.
2. In a bowl, place all ingredients except chocolate chips and lemon zest and beat until well combined.
3. Gently, fold in the chocolate chips and lemon zest.
4. Place ¼ of the mixture into preheated waffle iron and cook for about minutes or until golden brown.

5. Repeat with the remaining mixture.

6. Serve warm.

Nutrition: Calories: Net Carb: 1gFat: 4.8gSaturated Fat: 2.3gCarbohydrates: 1.5gDietary Fiber: 0.5g Sugar: 0.3gProtein: 4.3g

SAVORY CHAFFLES RECIPES

41. Vegan Chaffle

Preparation time: 5 minutes

Cooking Time: 25 Minutes

Ingredients:

- 1 Tbsp flaxseed meal
- 2 ½ Tbsp water
- ¼ cup low carb vegan cheese
- 2 Tbsp coconut flour
- 1 Tbsp low carb vegan cream cheese, softened
- Pinch of salt

Directions:

1. Turn on waffle maker to heat and oil it with cooking spray.
2. Mix flaxseed and water in a bowl. Leave for 5 minutes, until thickened and gooey.
3. Whisk remaining ingredients for chaffle.
4. Pour one half of the batter into the center of the waffle maker. Close and cook for 3-5 minutes.
5. Remove chaffle and serve.

Nutrition: Carbs: 33 g ;Fat: 25 g ;Protein: 25 g ;Calories: 450

42. Lemony Fresh Herbs Chaffles

Servings: 6

Cooking Time: 24 Minutes

Ingredients:

- ½ cup ground flaxseed
- 2 organic eggs
- ½ cup goat cheddar cheese, grated
- 2-4 tablespoons plain Greek yogurt
- 1 tablespoon avocado oil
- ½ teaspoon baking soda
- 1 teaspoon fresh lemon juice
- 2 tablespoons fresh chives, minced
- 1 tablespoon fresh basil, minced
- ½ tablespoon fresh mint, minced
- ¼ tablespoon fresh thyme, minced
- ¼ tablespoon fresh oregano, minced
- Salt and freshly ground black pepper, to taste

Directions:

1. Preheat a waffle iron and then grease it.

2. In a medium bowl, place all ingredients and with a fork, mix until well combined.

3. Divide the mixture into 6 portions.

4. Place 1 portion of the mixture into preheated waffle iron and cook for about minutes or until golden brown.

5. Repeat with the remaining mixture.

6. Serve warm.

Nutrition: Calories: 11et Carb: 0.9gFat: 7.9gSaturated Fat: 3gCarbohydrates: 3.7gDietary Fiber: 2.8g Sugar: 0.7gProtein: 6.4g

43. Italian Seasoning Chaffles

Preparation time: 6 minutes

Cooking Time: 8 Minutes

Servings: 2

Ingredients:

- ½ cup Mozzarella cheese, shredded

- 1 tablespoon Parmesan cheese, shredded

- 1 organic egg

- ¾ teaspoon coconut flour

- ¼ teaspoon organic baking powder

- 1/8 teaspoon Italian seasoning

- Pinch of salt

Directions:

1. Preheat a mini waffle iron and then grease it.

2. In a medium bowl, place all ingredients and with a fork, mix until well combined.

3. Place half of the mixture into preheated waffle iron and cook for about 4 minutes or until golden brown.

4. Repeat with the remaining mixture.

5. Serve warm.

Nutrition: Calories: 8et Carb: 1.9gFat: 5gSaturated Fat: 2.6gCarbohydrates: 3.8gDietary Fiber: 1.9g Sugar: 0.6gProtein: 6.5g

44. Basil Chaffles

Preparation time: 10 minutes

Cooking Time: 16 Minutes

Servings: 2

Ingredients:

- 2 organic eggs, beaten
- ½ cup Mozzarella cheese, shredded
- 1 tablespoon Parmesan cheese, grated
- 1 teaspoon dried basil, crushed
- Pinch of salt

Directions:

1. Preheat a mini waffle iron and then grease it.
2. In a medium bowl, place all ingredients and mix until well combined.
3. Place 1/of the mixture into preheated waffle iron and cook for about 3-4 minutes or until golden brown.
4. Repeat with the remaining mixture.
5. Serve warm.

Nutrition: Calories: Net Carb: 0.4gFat: 4.2gSaturated Fat: 1.6gCarbohydrates: 0.4gDietary Fiber: 0g Sugar: 0.2gProtein: 5.7g

45. <u>Bacon Chaffles</u>

Preparation time: 6 minutes

Cooking Time: 5 Minutes

Servings: 2

Ingredients:

- 2 eggs
- ½ cup cheddar cheese
- ½ cup mozzarella cheese
- ¼ tsp baking powder
- ½ Tbsp almond flour
- 1 Tbsp butter, for waffle maker
- For the filling:
- ¼ cup bacon, chopped
- 2 Tbsp green onions, chopped

Directions:

1. Turn on waffle maker to heat and oil it with cooking spray.
2. Add eggs, mozzarella, cheddar, almond flour, and baking powder to a blender and pulse 10 times, so cheese is still chunky.

3. Add bacon and green onions. Pulse 2-times to combine.

4. Add one half of the batter to the waffle maker and cook for 3 minutes, until golden brown.

5. Repeat with remaining batter.

6. Add your toppings and serve hot.

Nutrition: Carbs: 3 g ;Fat: 38 g ;Protein: 23 g ;Calories: 446

46. <u>Sausage Chaffles</u>

Preparation time: 5 minutes 2

Cooking Time: 1 Hour

Servings: 2

Ingredients:

- 1 pound gluten-free bulk Italian sausage, crumbled
- 1 organic egg, beaten
- 1 cup sharp Cheddar cheese, shredded
- ¼ cup Parmesan cheese, grated
- 1 cup almond flour
- 2 teaspoons organic baking powder

Directions:

1. Preheat a mini waffle iron and then grease it.
2. In a medium bowl, place all ingredients and with your hands, mix until well combined.
3. Place about 3 tablespoons of the mixture into preheated waffle iron and cook for about 3 minutes or until golden brown.
4. Carefully, flip the chaffle and cook for about 2 minutes or until golden brown.
5. Repeat with the remaining mixture.

6. Serve warm.

Nutrition: Calories: 238Net Carb: 1.2gFat: 19.6gSaturated Fat: 6.1gCarbohydrates: 2.2gDietary Fiber: 1g Sugar: 0.4gProtein: 10.8g

47. Scallion Cream Cheese Chaffle

Preparation time: 6 minutes

Cooking Time: 20 Minutes

Servings: 2

Ingredients:

- 1 large egg
- ½ cup of shredded mozzarella
- 2 Tbsp cream cheese
- 1 Tbsp everything bagel seasoning
- 1-2 sliced scallions

Directions:

1. Turn on waffle maker to heat and oil it with cooking spray.
2. Beat egg in a small bowl.
3. Add in ½ cup mozzarella.
4. Pour half of the mixture into the waffle maker and cook for 3-minutes.
5. Remove chaffle and repeat with remaining mixture.
6. Let them cool, then cover each chaffle with cream cheese, sprinkle with seasoning and scallions.

Nutrition: Carbs: 8 g ;Fat: 11 g ;Protein: 5 g ;Calories: 168

48. Broccoli Chaffles

Preparation time: 6 minutes

Cooking Time: 8 Minutes

Servings: 2

Ingredients:

- 1/3 cup raw broccoli, chopped finely
- ¼ cup Cheddar cheese, shredded
- 1 organic egg
- ½ teaspoons garlic powder
- ½ teaspoons dried onion, minced
- Salt and freshly ground black pepper, to taste

Directions:

1. Preheat a mini waffle iron and then grease it.
2. In a medium bowl, place all ingredients and, mix until well combined.
3. Place ¼ of the mixture into preheated waffle iron and cook for about 4 minutes or until golden brown.
4. Repeat with the remaining mixture.
5. Serve warm.

Nutrition: Calories: 9et Carb: 1.5gFat: 6.9gSaturated Fat: 3.7gCarbohydrates: 2gDietary Fiber: 0.5g Sugar: 0.7gProtein: 6.8g

49. Chicken Taco Chaffles

Preparation time: 6 minutes

Cooking Time: 8 Minutes

Servings: 2

Ingredients:

- 1/3 cup cooked grass-fed chicken, chopped
- 1 organic egg
- 1/3 cup Monterrey Jack cheese, shredded
- ¼ teaspoon taco seasoning

Directions:

1. Preheat a mini waffle iron and then grease it.
2. In a bowl, place all the ingredients and mix until well combined.
3. Place half of the mixture into preheated waffle iron and cook for about 4 minutes or until golden brown.
4. Repeat with the remaining mixture.
5. Serve warm.

Nutrition: Calories: 141Net Carb: 1.1gFat: 8.9gSaturated Fat: 4.9gCarbohydrates: 1.1gDietary Fiber: 0g Sugar: 0.2gProtein: 13.5g

50. Bacon & 3-cheese Chaffles

Preparation time: 10 minutes

Cooking Time: 8 Minutes

Servings: 2

Ingredients:

- 3 large organic eggs
- ½ cup Swiss cheese, grated
- 1/3 cup Parmesan cheese, grated
- 1/4 cup cream cheese, softened
- 4 tablespoons almond flour
- 1 tablespoon coconut flour
- ½ teaspoon onion powder
- ½ teaspoon garlic powder
- ½ teaspoon dried basil, crushed
- ½ teaspoon dried oregano, crushed
- ½ teaspoon organic baking powder
- Salt and freshly ground black pepper, to taste
- 4 cooked bacon slices, cut in half

Directions:

1. Preheat a waffle iron and then grease it.

2. In a bowl, place all the ingredients except for bacon and mix until well combined.

3. Place ¼ of the mixture into preheated waffle iron.

4. Arrange 2 halved bacon slices over mixture and cook for about 2 minutes or until golden brown.

5. Repeat with the remaining mixture and bacon slices.

6. Serve warm.

Nutrition: Calories: 259Net Carb: 3.2gFat: 20.1gSaturated Fat: 8.Carbohydrates: 4.8gDietary Fiber: 1.6g Sugar: 1gProtein: 13.9g

CONCLUSION

The most documented advantage of a keto diet is fast weight reduction. Counter to belief, many people have described becoming less hungry. As well as this, keto can minimize acne, and it may even boost cardiac protection and maintain neural activity, either way, you can contact a medical practitioner to get their opinions and guidelines once you start buying avocado crates and particularly if you have problems with obesity. The requirements of everyone are different and do not fit for you individually what works for the overwhelming majority of citizens. Apart from having an eye on the fat quality, when selecting food products, you can also evaluate the protein. In your keto diet, you just require moderate protein – around 20 percent of your total calorie consumption can come from proteins – and some nuts appear to be rich in protein.

From a mineral and vitamin standpoint, ensure fibrous fruits and vegetables such as cabbage, broccoli and cauliflower are integrated.

Getting into ketosis takes around 2-4 days (suggesting carbs are low enough) based on the person. Also, the carb content needed to achieve ketosis can differ between individuals. "Initial weight loss would be very swift but bear in mind that much of it will be contained in glycogen (carbs) and water. Afterward, slow weight loss will follow due to a calorie shortage and consuming more fat as a fuel". As the expression goes, slow and steady wins the race, and this is extremely valid for diets. You will easily lose weight on keto, but you may need to be vigilant with long-term results to help your body adapt to your new diet.

No doubt, chaffles dominated the world of low-carb: they are awesome. For unlimited combinations of seasoning, sweet or savory, you may add and alter using a very simple ingredient with just cheese and eggs. Use it individually or as the resource for seasonings and toppings. A simple calculation of the chaffle is 1/2 cup of 1 egg cheese for every chaffle. Commence adding coconut or almond flour. Check around with the cheeses. Add vegetables, berries, spices or nuts and let the imagination go away.

Chaffles can be frozen and processed, so a large proportion can be made and stored for quick and extremely fast meals. If you don't have a waffle maker, just cook the mixture like a pancake in a frying pan, or even cooler, in a fryer-pan. They won't get all the fluffy sides to achieve like you're using a waffle maker, but they're definitely going to taste great. Depending on which cheese you choose, the carbs and net calorie number can shift a little bit. However, in general, whether you use real, whole milk cheese, chaffles are completely carb-free. For up to a month, chaffles will be frozen. However, defrosting them absorbs plenty of moist, which makes it difficult to get their crisp again. Chaffles are rich in fat and moderate in protein and low in carb. Chaffle is a very well established and popular technique to hold people on board. And the chaffles are more durable and better than most forms of keto bread. "What a high-carb diet you may be desirous of. A nonstick waffle maker is something that makes life easier, and it's a trade-off that's happy to embrace for our wellbeing.

To sum up, the keto diet is healthy and helpful to your wellbeing and weight reduction if you are very diligent and conscious of it. The best way to monitor your keto commitment is to use a diet tracking app, where you will easily set the target amount of macronutrients / macro breakdown (on keto, it would most definitely be 75 percent fat, 5 percent carbohydrates and 20 percent protein) and check the labels of the food you choose to consume.

Over everything, as for any transition to lifestyle, permit yourself some time to acclimate. You'll see some fast changes almost instantly, but to hold the weight off, you'll have to stay with the plan, even if improvement slows down a little. Slowing down does not mean that the new diet has stopped working; it just means that the body is actually-adjusting itself to meet the new diet. Weight reduction, or something like losing the unnecessary excess weight, is just a side result of a healthy, better lifestyle that can support you in the long run and not only in the short term.